The Posturelate

Written by Dr. Andrew Buser, D.C., C.S.C.S.
& Markus Greus, P.T.

Illustrated by Andrew Buser, D.C., C.S.C.S.

Edited by Dr. M. Rhiannon Hutton, D.C., M.A.O.M.

Table of Contents

Introduction

In order to give the reader context, it is important to understand that the evolution of musculoskeletal therapies began thousands of years ago. Early modalities involved treatments of various forms, including movement, stretching and exercise, stimulation of various meridians, massage, and more. Recently, practitioners have explored the effectiveness of more focused goals. This includes, but is not limited to, the evaluation of moving bones to affect the nervous and lymphatic systems, myofascial release, activation and stability training, range of motion therapy, and skeletal realignment using active muscular engagement. Acknowledging the success of these therapies, we hope to add an important new element to the musculoskeletal practitioner's repertoire, the facilitation of, what we call the "Anti-Gravity Kinetic Chain." The "Anti-Gravity Kinetic Chain" is a soft-tissue chain comprised of muscles, ligaments, and fascia, which supports static and dynamic postural equilibrium through the primary actions of counteracting the affect of gravity on the body and stabilizing the origins of mover-muscles. Musculoskeletal therapies have evolved for thousands of years. Pioneers in these fields include ancient acupuncturists, masseurs, and yogis, Patanjali, Hippocrates, Galenus, Dr. Daniel David Palmer, Dr. George Goodheart, Dr. A.T. Still, Dr. Ida Rolf, F.M. Alexander, Moshé Feldenkrais, Dr. Vladimir Janda, Dr. William Sutherland, Joseph Pilates, Pete Egoscue, Robin McKenzie, Dr. Bess Mensendieck, and others. We invite theorists and researchers of all disciplines to explore these concepts and offer their ideas, whether or not they are consistent with our own.

Gravity/Antigravity Equilibrium as the Basis for Function, Dysfunction, and Compensation in Human Biomechanics

An examination of human posture texts reveals many different understandings of postural dysfunction. Surprisingly, few accounts offer a compelling description of what normal or optimal postural function looks like. We argue that this approach is backwards, as dysfunction cannot truly be understood until function has been defined and understood. Defining optimal postural function is no small task, as movement outcomes can be achieved through an almost endless variety of strategies, making it difficult to qualify one strategy as superior to another. Here we take a deductive approach to understanding human postural function, which we suggest must comply with some sort of survival algorithm. Though we allow for a degree of variation to accommodate adaptations to specific activity, we argue that optimal biomechanical function is uniform across the human species. To suggest that the human body does not operate according to a functional design which contains a primary biomechanical strategy would be to imply that the human genome is, at least to a degree, a product of chance. More likely is the case that evolution favored biomechanics and musculoskeletal morphologies that confer advantages for survival. Optimal movement strategies then, are those that maximize advantages for survival with a given set of resources.

Human movement is an act of manipulating the balance of applied and resistive forces to achieve a desired outcome. Of these forces, we must find ourselves in constant equilibrium with one force in particular, gravity.

2

Considering that the quintessential position of the human body is in an upright bipedal stance, function must primarily achieve equilibrium with gravity in this position. All higher order movement strategies must be conditioned on this design principle. Keep in mind that gravity does not disappear when we choose to move for a specific purpose like reaching for a glass. The following article details our model of human function based on the principle of optimizing the body's relationship with gravity in upright bipedal stance.

Posture in Theory and in Practice

The term "posture" conjures notions like joint stability, muscle balance, skeletal alignment, and neuromuscular control, concepts, which have meaning in both clinical and research domains. Widely varying interpretation of these concepts has lead to a general inconsistency with regard to exactly what posture is and how it works. The most popular theories make reference to "core" muscles surrounding the axial skeleton, which are understood to create stability during movement. Variations of this theory, which are scientifically viable, do not always pass muster in clinical practice. Similarly, valuable clinical models are not always supported by scientific data. The value of the scientific method cannot be overstated. We should not, however, limit our thinking to only that which is supported by experimental data. Research findings are constrained by laboratory technology and the difficulties associated with testing complex, multivariate hypotheses in a well-controlled setting. Because human movement science is so complex, observational approaches can make a valuable contribution to our knowledge base. This is nothing new. In fact, scientific investigation of human movement tends to be guided by clinical practice as much as by experimental data.

3

Equilibrium with Gravity in Upright Stance

On a fundamental level, it can be argued that evolution and the process of natural selection guide human form and function. To that end, the body has evolved to meet certain criteria that promote its own survival. Because resources like bone and muscle tissue are scarce, the human frame must be designed in such a way as to distribute strain efficiently. We also acknowledge that it must allow for range of motion, strength, speed, endurance, and so forth, factors, which may not always complement one another on a design level. In studies of posture and movement, metabolic expenditure is often used as a proxy for efficiency.[1,2] In the task of static bipedal standing, metabolic expenditure will be minimized to the extent that its load-bearing sites maintain proximity to the Line of Gravity. Such a posture would theoretically reduce the moments, and therefore counter-moments, about these load-bearing joints that occur due to the force of gravity.[3] Sven Carlsöö proposed, as early as 1961 that "prime postural muscles" should be considered those involved in resisting the effect of gravity.[4] This, we argue, is the most fundamental concept in human posture—both static and dynamic. As, the role of human muscle in stabilizing against any force must ultimately be founded upon its function in stabilizing against gravity.

The location of the Line of Gravity (LOG), as it falls in standing posture, in the sagittal plane carries important implications for theories of posture and equilibrium. Research has presented us with varying accounts of its location under a number of experimental manipulations.[5-8] We begin with the sagittal plane, as it is the primary plane of movement and the plane in which we position ourselves

4

for most of our daily activities. While our accounts diverge in some areas, we have found that Levangie & Norkin's[9] summary most closely approximates our observation and seems to be the most clinically applicable. Given the position of the Line of Gravity in their model, it follows that the skeleton will collapse in the sagittal plane under gravity according to the patterns depicted in the list below. These patterns are largely based on the work of Levangie & Norkin [9], with respect to the spatial position of bones and joints, and upon the generally corroborating work of Myers,[10] with respect to identifying groups or lines of muscles that perform a united task. It is also of note that the Line of Gravity does not pass directly through the center of the skeletal load-bearing sites as the vast majority of contemporary theories postulate. This is an important distinction in our understanding for multiple reasons. First, this arrangement facilitates loading into soft, elastic tissue rather than loading into structures more susceptible to deformation. More importantly, however, it implies the existence of, what we refer to as, a specific "collapsing tendency" of the skeleton, both spatial and angular. For instance, under gravity the knee joint will move forward in space and hyperextend. We also propose that it will also abduct and rotate internally, as will be discussed below.

Figures 1 and 2: Current mainstream theory of the body's stabilizing measures in response to the affects of gravity.

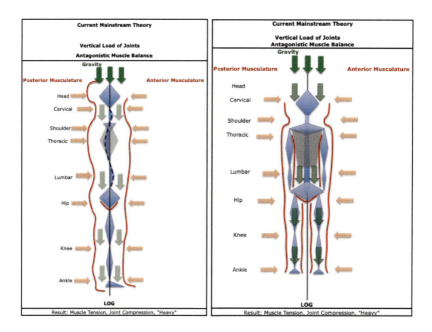

Gravitational "Collapsing Tendencies" of the Skeleton During Static Standing in the Sagittal Plane (Figure 3)

- Ankle: Dorsiflexion (The tibia, fibula and talus translate anteriorly over a supposed fixed calcaneus.)
- Tibia/Fibula: Internal/medial rotation of tibia, anterior translation and abduction of proximal ends.
- Knee: Anterior/forward deviation relative to ankle with hyperextension, varus stress, and internal rotation.
- Femur: Internal, medial rotation, anterior translation relative to the tibia, and abduction of the distal ends.
- Hip: Anterior/forward deviation relative to knee and lumbar spine, internal/medial rotation, abduction, hyperextension; Unilateral weakness would yield contralateral pelvic rotation.
- Pelvis/SI: Posterior tilt/flexion (The pelvis deviates forward relative to LOG; the iliac crest, however, collapses posteriorly to the acetabulum.)
- Lumbosacral Spine: Flexion (Sacral counter-nutation if the pelvis remains fixed, lumbar spine flexion); Unilateral weakness would yield ipsilateral rotation and ipsilateral lateral flexion/ deviation of the vertebrae to the side opposite the weakness.
- Shoulder: "Tipping" forward (Scapular protraction/abduction, scapular winging, scapular downward rotation, humeral internal rotation.)
- Thoracic Spine: Flexion; Unilateral weakness yields ipsilateral rotation and ipsilateral lateral flexion / lateral deviation of the vertebrae to the side opposite the weakness.
- Cervical Spine: Flexion; Unilateral weakness yields ipsilateral rotation and ipsilateral lateral flexion / lateral deviation of the vertebrae to the side opposite the weakness.

- Head: Forward deviation relative to spine, rearward deviation relative to ankle, downward gaze, lateral deviation of the head to the side opposite the weakness.

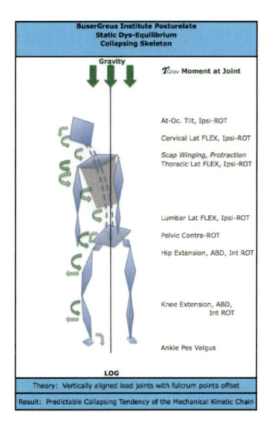

Figure 3: The BuserGreus Model demonstrating the affect of gravity on the skeleton.

With regard to the above, and specifically the feet, in the coronal plane, we have left out the abduction/adduction translation "collapsing tendency" for the following reason:

In the snapshot of a single moment in time where the body is receiving feedback from joint and muscle proprioceptors

8

and in turn reacting with continuous feed-forward regulatory stimulus to mitigate the momentary collapsing of the skeleton, the feet are most typically affixed to the ground, as in static posture or the stance phase of gait. That is, the static friction force of the ground-foot interface provides for inhibition of momentary abduction or adduction translation of the foot upon the ground. Thus, in this model, as the proposed postural chain progressively weakens, the foot, which consists of the calcaneus, metatarsals and phalanges which are in contact with the ground, and sometimes the tarsal bones (in pes planus) is therefore assumed to remain static with regards to coronal translation of abduction or adduction due to this inherent frictional force. This gives a point of relativity for comparison of all other joints. All joints collapse around the feet in one direction or another when during a state of pure postural chain weakness. Following such weakness where the body is able to sense and adjust to its now unstable Center of Gravity (COG), it often is observed clinically to be followed by numerous compensatory measures to re-stabilize in spite of the dysfunction in the postural chain. At this point the feet often splay outward, rotate inward, widen or narrow in stance, or stagger stance. These compensatory measures involve recruitment of more superficial muscle groups as will be discussed later in the article. For now, it should be understood that our model, above, reflects a snapshot in time during static posture with weakness in the postural muscles, which results in the skeleton collapsing around a relatively fixed foot.

The Basis for Biomechanical Function

Extending Carlsöö's notion of a related collection of primary postural muscles should first meet the criteria of resisting these collapsing tendencies. Ideally, they will resist gravity in a given area without contributing to its effects elsewhere. For example, the hamstring group, a popular candidate for

postural maintenance in many theories, opposes ext
at the knee but accentuates gravity-induced hip exte
and posterior pelvic tilt, which argues against its function as
a "postural" muscle. There does, however, exist a chain of
fascially continuous muscles that appears well suited to
address the body's anti-gravity needs. Myers[10] describes
the Deep Front Line(DFL) which travels from foot to head
along the surface of skeleton. With certain modifications to
Myers' DFL line, based upon our clinical observations, we
have arrived at an integrated chain of muscles that tends to
distract joints. This "distracting tendency" is based on the
morphology of each joint and counteracting the effects of
gravity. We refer to this integrated chain of muscles as the
Antigravity Kinetic Chain[TM] (AGKC). Appropriately, the
muscles that constitute the AGKC, as well as many in
Myers' DFL, tend to lack perfect antagonists. That is,
muscles that simultaneously oppose their effects in all
three planes. Their most complete antagonist, it would
seem, is gravity itself. This agonist/antagonist relationship
is important, as it allows for a definition of stability that does
not require co-activation of agonist/antagonist muscle
groups as argued in other theories. There may be
situations in which a co-activation strategy is appropriate
for additional stability; however, such a strategy would
generally lead to increased compressive forces and
metabolic expenditure. Any co-activation during normal
static standing should therefore be minimal. In the context
of postural static equilibrium, the forces we should be most
concerned with are gravity, an external force, and that
which opposes it from within.

Muscles of the Anti-Gravity Kinetic Chain^{TM} (Figure 6)

- Foot: Tibialis posterior
- Ankle: Tibialis posterior
- Lower leg: Tibialis posterior
- Knee: Popliteus
- Femur: Adductors minimus, brevis, longus, and magnus; pectineus, iliacus, psoas
- Hip: Iliacus, psoas, pectineus
- Pelvis/SI: Iliacus, psoas, pectineus, quadratus lumborum, multifidi, internal abdominal oblique
- Lumbar Spine: Quadratus lumborum, serratus posterior inferior, psoas, rotators, levatores costarum, semispinales, multifidi
- Thoracic Spine: Diaphragm, rhomboids, serratus posterior superior, lower internal obliques, rotators, levatores costarum, semispinales
- Shoulder: Inferior rhomboid, serratus anterior
- Cervical Spine: Scalenes, longus colli, sternohyoid, sternothyroid, thyrohyoid, omohyoid, rotators, levatores costarum, semispinales
- Head: Longus capitus, scalenes, sternocleidomastoid

Having multi-planar lines of action, the muscles of the AGKC can be used to extrapolate transverse and frontal plane gravitational collapsing tendencies of the skeleton in upright bipedal stance. A complete, multi-planar list of these collapsing tendencies follows. Although extrapolating transverse and frontal plane collapsing tendencies from the muscles identified as Anti-Gravitational in the sagittal plane may at first appear circular, we contend that the factors we have already outlined which support the AGKC's postural role provide a sufficient theoretical basis for doing so. The most important of these factors are, fascial continuity, non-interference with other links in the chain, and lack of direct internal antagonists. Furthermore, while we invite scrutiny from other practitioners, we emphasize the clinical value of this model, which has been derived over the course of thousands of patient treatments. Having discussed the hamstrings as unsuitable in supporting postural alignment, now consider the iliopsoas. Under gravity, we observe internal rotation, abduction, and hyperextension of the hip; forward translation and posterior tilt of the pelvis; and flexion of the lumbar spine. The iliopsoas and adductor group resist all "collapsing tendencies" of the skeleton without the need for muscular activation of the abdominals, hamstrings, rectus femoris, or gluteals.

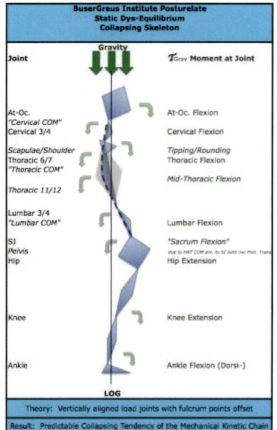

Figure 4: The BuserGreus Model demonstrating the affect of gravity on the skeleton in the sagittal plane.

13

Figure 5: The BuserGreus Model of the affect of gravity on the skeleton and the soft tissues of the AGKC in the sagittal plane.

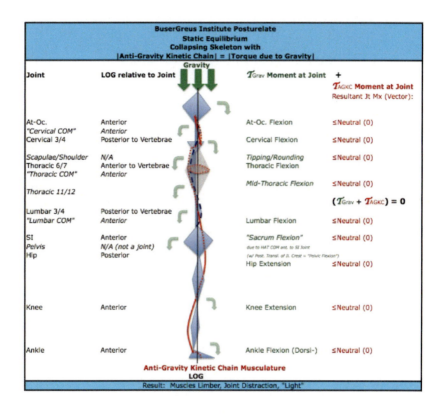

Figure 6: The BuserGreus Model of the affect of the AGKC in response to gravity in the sagittal plane.

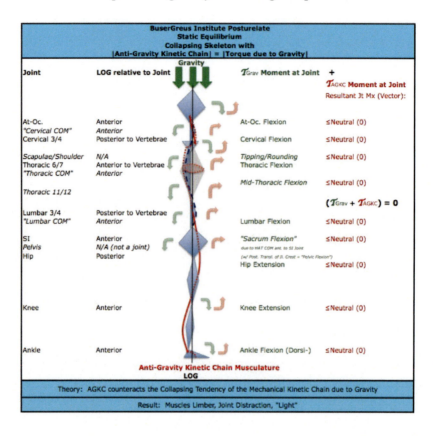

The table within the figure reads:

BuserGreus Institute Posturelate
Static Equilibrium
Collapsing Skeleton with
|Anti-Gravity Kinetic Chain| = |Torque due to Gravity|

Joint	LOG relative to Joint	Gravity	T_{Grav} Moment at Joint	+ T_{AGKC} Moment at Joint — Resultant Jt Mx (Vector):
At-Oc.	Anterior		At-Oc. Flexion	≤Neutral (0)
"Cervical COM"	Anterior			
Cervical 3/4	Posterior to Vertebrae		Cervical Flexion	≤Neutral (0)
Scapulae/Shoulder	N/A		Tipping/Rounding	≤Neutral (0)
Thoracic 6/7	Anterior to Vertebrae		Thoracic Flexion	
"Thoracic COM"	Anterior			
			Mid-Thoracic Flexion	≤Neutral (0)
Thoracic 11/12				
				$(T_{Grav} + T_{AGKC}) = 0$
Lumbar 3/4	Posterior to Vertebrae			
"Lumbar COM"	Anterior		Lumbar Flexion	≤Neutral (0)
SI	Anterior		"Sacrum Flexion"	≤Neutral (0)
Pelvis	N/A (not a joint)		due to HAT COM ant. to SI Joint	
Hip	Posterior		(w/ Post. Transl. of Il. Crest = "Pelvic Flexion")	
			Hip Extension	≤Neutral (0)
Knee	Anterior		Knee Extension	≤Neutral (0)
Ankle	Anterior		Ankle Flexion (Dorsi-)	≤Neutral (0)

Anti-Gravity Kinetic Chain Musculature
LOG

Theory: AGKC counteracts the Collapsing Tendency of the Mechanical Kinetic Chain due to Gravity

Result: Muscles Limber, Joint Distraction, "Light"

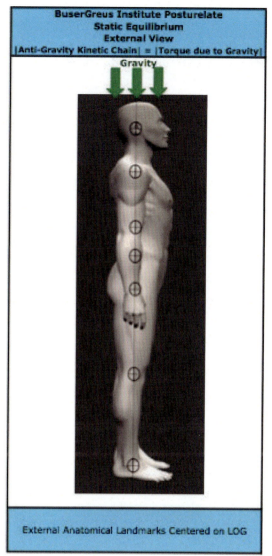

BuserGreus Institute Posturelate
Static Equilibrium
External View
|Anti-Gravity Kinetic Chain| = |Torque due to Gravity|
Gravity

External Anatomical Landmarks Centered on LOG

Figure 7: Notice that the Line of Gravity, as viewed from outside of the body, still appears consistent with the contemporary clinical model.

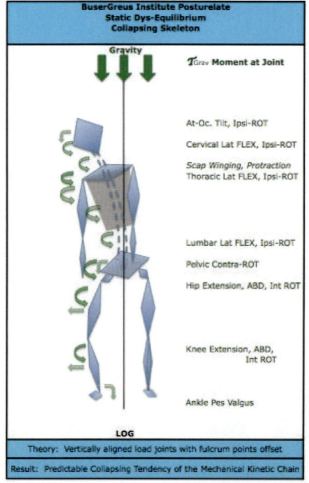

Figure 8: The BuserGreus Model of the affect of gravity on the skeleton in the sagittal plane.

Figure 9: The BuserGreus Model of the affect of the AGKC in response to gravity in the coronal plane.

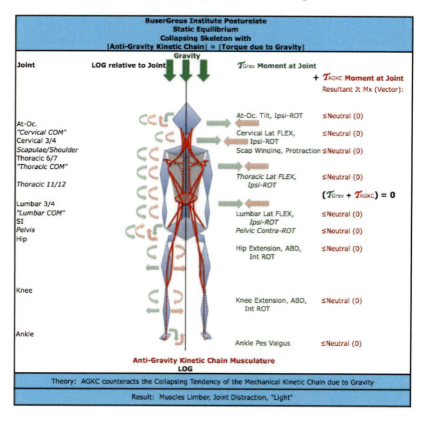

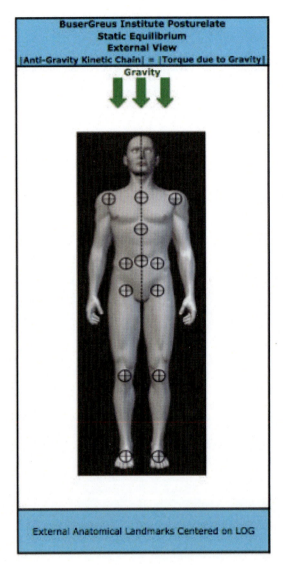

BuserGreus Institute Posturelate
Static Equilibrium
External View
|Anti-Gravity Kinetic Chain| = |Torque due to Gravity|

Gravity

External Anatomical Landmarks Centered on LOG

Figure 10: The Line of Gravity as viewed from outside of the body. Notice this view still appears consistent with the contemporary clinical model.

Gravitational "Collapsing Tendencies" of the Skeleton During Static Standing in All Planes

- Foot: Pronation/Eversion with collapsed arch/pes planus.
- Ankle: Dorsiflexion (tibia and talus travels/translates forward over foot/calcaneus), pes valgus.
- Tibia/Fibula: Internal/medial rotation of tibia, anterior translation and abduction of proximal ends
- Knee: Anterior/forward deviation relative to ankle with hyperextension, varus stress, and internal rotation.
- Femur: Internal, medial rotation, anterior translation relative to the tibia, and abduction of the distal ends.
- Hip: Anterior/forward deviation relative to knee and lumbar spine, internal/medial rotation, abduction, hyperextension; Unilateral weakness would yield contralateral pelvic rotation (i.e. Right AGKC weakness at the level of the right hip will cause the right hip to translate forward relative to the left, or left pelvic rotation.)
- Pelvis/SI: Posterior tilt/flexion (The pelvis deviates forward relative to LOG; the iliac crest, however, collapses posteriorly to the acetabulum); Unilateral weakness of the AGKC at this level (i.e. iliacus, iliopsoas, and quadratus lumborum oblicuus), and/or a right versus left innominate bone disparity in the sagittal plane would yield contralateral pelvic rotation. Remember that rotation in the transverse plane is often due to unilateral translation in the sagittal plane.
- Lumbosacral Spine: Lumbar and sacral flexion (sacral counter-nutation due to the breakdown of functional SI biomechanics); Unilateral weakness would yield ipsilateral sacral/vertebral posterior rotation, and ipsilateral lateral flexion accompanied

by lateral deviation of the vertebrae to the side opposite the weakness.

- Shoulder: "Tipping" forward (arm extension, scapular protraction/abduction, scapular winging, scapular downward rotation, humeral internal rotation.)
- Thoracic Spine: Flexion; Unilateral weakness yields ipsilateral rotation and ipsilateral lateral flexion/lateral deviation of the vertebrae to the side opposite the weakness.
- Cervical Spine: Flexion; unilateral weakness yields ipsilateral rotation and ipsilateral lateral flexion/lateral deviation of the vertebrae to the side opposite the weakness.
- Head: Forward deviation relative to spine, rearward deviation relative to ankle, downward gaze/lateral deviation of the head to the side opposite the weakness.

Facilitating the AGKC therapeutically is often associated with the feeling of "lightness." We refer to this as the "Antigravity Feeling" and use this sensation as a subjective measure to evaluate static and dynamic posture as well as check the effectiveness of our interventions. This phenomenon is likely related to antigravity mechanics and optimization of lever systems throughout the body. As an example, the psoas is better suited than the rectus femoris to prevent the hip and pelvis from collapsing under gravity in standing posture, as it is the deepest and most closely related to the articular surface.

While this feeling is most readily understood as a biomechanical phenomenon, we believe there to be additional contributing factors. Neurologically, a limited conscious experience of the work of postural equilibrium may relate to cerebellar- and vestibular-driven processes that regulate posture and origin stability.[11] Additionally, antigravity muscles should consist primarily of stam oriented fibers, possibly contributing to a metabolic advantage. Some investigations would support this theory with regard to the psoas.[12,13] To test this metabolic advantage, try standing with your abdominals, gluteals, or quadriceps engaged and experience how quickly fatigue and discomfort set in. In comparison to the muscles of the AGKC, which should reflect a high capacity for slow-twitch engagement and aerobic endurance. Much of the stabilization they provide is likely derived from an elastic component rather than voluntary contraction.

We propose, maintaining static postural equilibrium is the primary responsibility of the AGKC. Under normal circumstances, only work beyond the maintenance of static posture or steady-state gait should require recruitment of additional muscle groups. This recruitment would ideally follow a progressive pattern from the deeper to the more superficial muscle layers as the level of demand increases. This hierarchical attendance to physical demands appears to be reflected in the body's hardwiring, wherein higher-level nerve roots often innervate deeper muscle layers. Nerve roots spawned from the spinal cord earlier than those innervating more superficial muscles within a given muscle compartment.

Figure 11: A comparison of the current Line of Gravity versus the Line of Gravity in the BuserGreus Model.

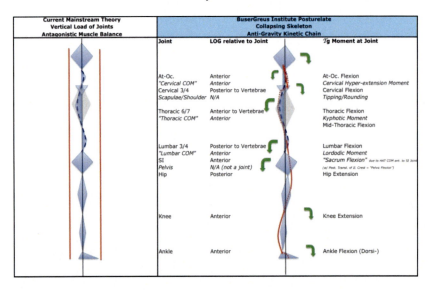

Current Mainstream Theory Vertical Load of Joints Antagonistic Muscle Balance	BuserGreus Institute Posturelate Collapsing Skeleton Anti-Gravity Kinetic Chain		
	Joint	LOG relative to Joint	*Tg* Moment at Joint
	At-Oc.	Anterior	At-Oc. Flexion
	"Cervical COM"	Anterior	Cervical Hyper-extension Moment
	Cervical 3/4	Posterior to Vertebrae	Cervical Flexion
	Scapulae/Shoulder	N/A	Tipping/Rounding
	Thoracic 6/7	Anterior to Vertebrae	Thoracic Flexion
	"Thoracic COM"	Anterior	Kyphotic Moment
			Mid-Thoracic Flexion
	Lumbar 3/4	Posterior to Vertebrae	Lumbar Flexion
	"Lumbar COM"	Anterior	Lordodic Moment
	SI	Anterior	"Sacrum Flexion" *due to HAT COM ant. to SI Joint*
	Pelvis	N/A (not a joint)	*(ie) Post. Transl. of B. Crest = "Pelvic Flexitor")*
	Hip	Posterior	Hip Extension
	Knee	Anterior	Knee Extension
	Ankle	Anterior	Ankle Flexion (Dorsi-)

Although in the depiction above, the exact center of the anatomic joint is not centered on the Line of Gravity, from the perspective of the observer upon a human model, the joints would appear "centered." The apices of the geometric representations of the above diagram are used to depict the fulcrum point within the joint, which is known to be askew from the anatomic center point based on each joint's morphology.

Biomechanical Dysfunction and Compensation

Superficial muscles can, however, be recruited "out of sequence" to assist, or take over, when the primary Anti-Gravity Kinetic Chain breaks down. This brings us to another key concept, the distinction between postural muscle dysfunction and superficial muscle compensation. To maximize the effect of any therapeutic strategy, we contend that the primary cause of misalignment,

23

dysfunction in the primary postural stabilizer chain, the AGKC must be addressed. For practical purposes, any postural deviation in the direction of the collapsing tendency of the skeleton can be understood to indicate an Anti-Gravity or postural-muscle dysfunction. Alternatively, deviations from proper alignment in directions inconsistent with the collapsing tendency indicate superficial muscular tension and should be understood as compensatory adaptations. These adaptations may mask weakness in the Anti-Gravity Chain, but their presence indicates that the primary mechanisms for alignment have broken down. Dysfunction would most often result from AGKC inhibition, denervation (i.e. lower motor neuron lesion), hypotonicity, weakness, metabolic deficiency, or maladaptive lengthening. This "dysfunction" is less a reflection of the "strength" of these muscles, in the traditional sense, and more so, an indication of loss of the sensitivity and adaptability of the chain of muscles to respond to their environment.

Two special cases should be noted in which the difference between dysfunction and compensation can be obscured. First, the AGKC can in rare cases become dysfunctionally short or tight (i.e. hyper-facilitated, hypertonic, inordinately strong, maladaptively short, or disinhibited as in the case of an upper motor neuron lesion). In this case, deviation should occur opposite the direction of skeletal collapsing. The second special case is more common and occurs following injury. Here, the AGKC may self-inhibit on the side of injury in an effort to "off-load" the damaged tissue. The contralateral AGKC, as well as the potential superficial muscles, work to pull the center of gravity to the uninjured side or change movement patterns to minimize stress to the involved tissues. This appears to be related to an attempt in the body to facilitate the healing process and prevent further injury.

As we mentioned, it is fitting that these compensatory backup systems exist. In earlier times they may have saved a human from the elements after he or she suffered an injury in the wilderness. Today they enable us to live our lives relatively undisturbed should something go wrong. Much like efficient strain distribution would promote human survival, so do the redundant systems that support posture and movement. Unfortunately, these compensatory systems appear to be playing an ever-increasing role in human movement. As technology replaces physical work and eliminates the need for humans to resist gravity actively, the ability to do so is becoming increasingly rare. While new technology may enhance quality of life on some levels, it does so at a considerable cost.

Dysfunction, Compensation, & Pain

When the ability to maintain an appropriate posture breaks down, our body lets us know. It does this out of necessity. Whether or not we are aware of any deficits in posture, there will most often be

Figure 12: A Collapsing Lumbo-pelvic tendency, indicated by the green arrow, with Thoracic Compensatory measures.

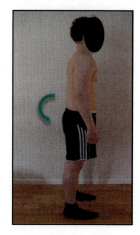

some form of pain as tissue damage reaches a critical extent. Here, pain can be understood as another means of supporting survival. If one were to place his/her hand on a hot stove inadvertently, pain would warn that person to remove the hand before it was destroyed. With chronic musculoskeletal pain the body may be signaling inefficiency in movement or stance, risk of injury, or degeneration of body segments

(Figure 12). Of course, we acknowledge that pain can stem from non-mechanical sources as well. We emphasize the need to rule out clinical red flags such as cancer and visceral referred pain with the assistance of a medical practitioner with a license to diagnose.

Understanding this relationship between posture and pain, the significance of the location of the Line of Gravity and the presence of the Anti-Gravity Kinetic Chain should be clear. When the body is meeting its operational goals there should not be a need, aside from traumatic injury, for pain in order to alert us that something is not functioning properly on a biomechanical level. It is our contention that proper facilitation of the Anti-Gravity Kinetic Chain —the true postural chain or "core"—can address a multitude of chronic musculoskeletal pain syndromes. As the strain of gravity is redistributed according to the body's design, gravitational moments about the skeleton will be minimized and no one segment or muscle will be required to take on more than its intended share of the load. Posture and locomotor activities will become coordinated, effortless, and natural rather than clumsy, lethargic, strenuous, and heavy. Joint position will be optimized and origins will be appropriately stabilized for movement. This, we argue, is the basis for biomechanical function and the appropriate context in which to describe the quality of an individual's movement behaviors.

Summary of Key Points

- Adequately describing postural dysfunction requires a model of optimal postural behavior.
- To understand function, we must identify a biologically adaptive equilibrium with gravity in upright bipedal stance.
- In upright bipedal stance, the human skeleton collapses according to a predetermined pattern.
- A muscle chain, the Anti-Gravity Kinetic Chain, exists to resist these tendencies. This chain is fascially continuous, does not interfere with itself, and appears to maintain an agonist/antagonist relationship with gravity.
- Movement behaviors are "functional" to the extent that they work within the blueprint of this relationship with gravity.
- A breakdown in the Anti-Gravity muscle chain constitutes a (primary) dysfunction.
- This can be seen as deviation from postural alignment in the direction of the "collapsing tendency" of the skeleton.
- Superficial muscular activity may compensate for these (primary) dysfunctions.
- This can be seen as deviation from postural alignment in a direction inconsistent with the "collapsing tendency" of the skeleton.

Chapter References

1.   Rubini A, Paoli A, Parmagnani A. Body metabolic rate and electromyographic activities of antigravitational muscles in supine and standing postures. European Journal of Applied Physiology. 2012;112(6):2045-2050.

2.   Saha D, Gard S, Fatone S, Ondra S. The effect of trunk-flexed postures on balance and metabolic energy expenditure during standing. Spine. 2007;32(15):1605-1611.

3.   Helmuth H. Biomechanics, evolution and upright stature. Anthropologischer Anzeiger. 1985;43(1):1-9.

4.   Carlsoo S. The static muscle load in different work positions: an electromyographic study. Ergonomics Ergonomics. 1961;4(3):193-211.

5.   Fox MG, Young OG. Placement of the gravital line in antero-posterior standing posture. Research Quarterly. American Association for Health, Physical Education and Recreation. 1954;25(3):277-285.

6.   Gangnet N, Pomero V, Dumas R, Skalli W, Vital JM. Variability of the spine and pelvis location with respect to the gravity line: a three-dimensional stereoradiographic study using a force platform. Surgical and radiologic anatomy. 2003;25(5-6):424-433.

7.   Pearsali DJ, Reid JG. Line of gravity relative to upright vertebral posture. Clinical Biomechanics Clinical Biomechanics. 1992;7(2):80-86.

8.   Schwab F, Lafage V, Boyce R, Skalli W, Farcy JP. Gravity line analysis in adult volunteers: age-related correlation with spinal parameters, pelvic parameters, and fool position. Spine. 2006;31(25):959-967.

9.   Levangie PK, Norkin CC. Joint structure and function: a comprehensive analysis. 2005: 493.

10.   Myers TW. Anatomy trains: myofascial meridians for manual and movement therapists. Elsevier Health Sciences; 2009:191-220.

11. Waxman SG. Clinical neuroanatomy. New York: Lange Medical Books/McGraw-Hill, Medical Pub. Division; 2003.

12. Kimura T. Composition of psoas major muscle fibers compared among humans, orangutans, and monkeys. Zeitschrift für Morphologie und Anthropologie. 2002;83(2/3):305-314.

13. Arbanas J, Klasan GS, Nikolic M, Jerkovic R, Miljanovic I, Malnar D. Fibre type composition of the human psoas major muscle with regard to the level of its origin. Journal of anatomy. 2009;215(6):636-641.

The BuserGreus Model of Postural Therapy: Principles-of-Therapy, Priorities-of-Work, & Evaluation of the Kinetic Chain

BuserGreus postural therapy practitioners achieve their goals through exercise. Though the therapy may seem to be strictly exercise-based, it is actually one's adherence to the logical flow of work that determines whether a successful strategy will be identified. In our case, these strategies take the form of corrective exercise sequences. However exercise, is merely one of many potential options for creating postural change. In the same way that a person can get from point A to point B using different forms of transportation, a postural therapist can arrive at his or her goal using different techniques. The flow of logic is like the route one must take to arrive at the final destination. Exercise just so happens to be our therapeutic "vehicle."

Here we describe what we refer to as the BuserGreus "Priorities-of-Work" and "Principles-of-Therapy". The Priorities-of-Work can be applied to select a suitable intervention strategy to promote advancement to the next phase of postural therapy. The Principles-of-Therapy outline a series of points along a progression toward postural integration, each of which must be met before procceding to the next. This is the progression that should be followed during the course of postural integration training.

The Priorities-of-Work: Load, Joint Mechanics, and Muscle Facilitation/Inhibition

Based on these theories, we regard postural dysfunction and the pain associated with it, to be primarily problems of a muscular/fascial origin as opposed to a skeletal, articular, or neurological origin. We certainly acknowledge that muscular dysfunction is not the only possible cause of postural misalignment, but contend that it is the most frequent and therefore the most relevant to this discussion. While this concept is applied in many existing forms of therapy, we add certain guidelines that we have found to be critical for any intervention to restore postural muscle function. These are the Priorities-of-Work. Briefly stated, the Priorities-of-Work dictate that the postural therapist must address load, joint mechanics, and muscle facilitation/inhibition, in that order, if the therapy is to be successful, efficient, and sustainable.

Load and joint mechanics are often confused. While they are related, they operate somewhat independently and must be addressed as independent phenomena. Load, refers to a weight-bearing joint's position in space relative to other weight-bearing joints (i.e. the atlanto-occipital joint relative to the shoulder, the sacroiliac joint relative to the hip, the knee, and the ankle). If a joint is properly aligned with respect to other joint(s), we refer to this segment as being "loaded." A loaded segment has mitigated the largest contributor to adverse lever moment arm contribution, the Torque due to Gravity. In addition to its position in space, each joint may be described in terms of its articular functions. When describing the load of a joint, we describe its load as in-line with, forward of, or behind other joints. And we describe its joint mechanics as flexed, extended/hyperextended, or neutral. Frontal or transverse planar load and joint mechanics should be described as well. These two factors, along with specific muscle facilitation or inhibition, may be adjusted to create an environment in which the Anti-Gravity Kinetic Chain (AGKC) can regain its ability to stabilize. Identifying and applying the combination of load, joint mechanics, and muscle facilitation/inhibition that will allow for stability of the AGKC, is the key to postural therapy.

To employ these concepts therapeutically, a practitioner should first select a position that his/her client can assume functionally. For example, a client that exhibits significant "collapsing tendencies" while standing might be better suited to begin his/her work in a supine position or, a position with less demand on the Anti-Gravity Chain. They may also require an external reference to assist him/her in finding a "loaded" position. For example, if the patient were supine, his reference would be the floor. Once an appropriate position is found, specific joint mechanics can be selected. In the case of a client collapsing under gravity without any superficial muscle compensation, we may wish to facilitate hip flexion and pelvic extension. Only after load and joint mechanics are addressed should we consider specific muscle activity. Continuing with the example, we could employ a variety of muscular forces to elicit a stabilizing response from the antigravity kinetic chain. As an example at this phase of therapy, when focusing on the AGKC function at the pelvis and hip, we might use gluteal squeezes to challenge the iliopsoas/quadratus lumborum to provide stability against the force of the gluteus maximus.

It may at first seem contradictory to place muscle facilitation/inhibition last on the list of priorities, given our position that postural integrity is primarily a muscular phenomenon. If the muscles are the problem, why not use them to affect load rather than bothering with load and joint mechanics first? This brings us to an important concept in posture and postural therapy, an idea we refer to as the "postural challenge." We view the Anti-Gravity Chain primarily as a collection of stabilizer-muscles rather than one of mover-muscles. That is, these muscles are primarily involved in opposing gravity and supporting more superficial muscles by assisting in stabilizing the origin of superficial/mover muscles, as opposed to creating movement themselves. Training or retraining the ability to stabilize should not be a matter of recruiting the stabilizer-muscle directly or consciously, per se. Instead, we should seek to recruit these muscles in their capacity as stabilizers against gravity and other more conscious muscle actions. To do this, we must find the positions and actions that will require a stabilization response. Further, we must do so without exceeding the capacity of the Anti-Gravity Chain. Otherwise, the work is rerouted to one of the suboptimal backup systems, or systems that tend to dominate given the prevailing conditions in most bodies. The stabilization required by a given position or exercise is its postural challenge. Postural challenges are met by muscles, but not by mover-muscles. Rather, we use direct conscious recruitment, or inhibition, of muscles in their "mover" roles to elicit a subconscious stabilizing response from the AGKC. This direct recruitment/inhibition of mover-muscles is a tertiary consideration in creating this subconscious, stabilizing response in a therapeutic environment. In order for the appropriate muscles to rise to the postural challenge, proper load and joint mechanics must first be in place.

The priority-of-work flow is exceedingly simple, but its effects are profound and should always guide intervention. Knowing that musculoskeletal dysfunction is a whole-body, multi-system phenomenon and not something that occurs in isolation, it is best to approach it as such. Addressing muscle length or articular dynamics is not likely to succeed if the joints are not first restored to their proper positions in space relative to one another. We have seen empirically that lower-order problems in the Priorities-of-Work continuum are often resolved without any direct attention. For example, persistent muscle tension is commonly relieved when load is reestablished. Conversely, we do not observe the opposite to be true. That is, despite tireless attention focused on muscles or joint mechanics, such as directly stretching the hamstrings, load is rarely achieved by working on these alone, and any lasting effect on these entities is often elusive.

Principles-of-Therapy

- Reduce the strain. Research has demonstrated that pain affects motor control.[1-3] We have observed that pain signals and sub-pain threshold tissue damage signals from the body to the central nervous system will result in subconscious compensatory responses to offload the sight of injury. Even when the patient is unaware of injury and without conscious pain, typical biomechanical compensation patterns can be observed. The system's priority, in this case, is not efficient load distribution, but rather to protect and heal the painful area. The Anti-Gravity Chain will be shut down in favor of whichever backup strategy best addresses these new demands. In this phase, clients should be placed in positions that unload strained areas. Additionally, alignment should be promoted to the extent permitted by the pain to ensure functional orientation of new tissue.
- Connect the kinetic chain. As will be discussed later, the kinetic chain is the mechanism whereby the body transmits and distributes strain with maximal efficiency. It also allows forces to be communicated from segment to segment during movement. Reestablishing this connection is necessary to ensure that the Anti-Gravity muscles are free to stabilize against gravity and against

34

mover-muscles in both static and in dynamic posture.

- Build on existing function. As will also be further elaborated, it is necessary to create the conditions under which the Anti-Gravity Chain becomes the most logical choice for maintaining posture. Otherwise, the assignment will go to another collection of muscles, which will ultimately perpetuate some degree of dysfunction/compensation. With this in mind, we must be careful not to ask so much of the Anti-Gravity Chain that it is incapable of rising to the occasion without assistance from superficial muscle chains. The existing level of function among the Anti-Gravity muscles will dictate our therapeutic starting point. The best strategy is to note the level of function then set the stage for the chain to expand its role gradually. For example, if the client is loaded bilaterally at the ankle, knee, and hip, we might begin with a position that provides some assistance to the remaining load joints, such as the sacroiliac, spine, shoulders, and head, before challenging them under more demanding conditions. This might be thought of as learning to ride a bike with training wheels before attempting the real thing.
- Promote symmetry and load. As the body graduates to accommodate higher levels of postural demand, the goal is to achieve a level of function in which each of the load joints assumes its natural/ optimal position with respect to the Line of Gravity. Here it may be said that the body is "loaded," which is a good indication that the Anti-Gravity Chain is strong. Compensatory chains can approximate the "loaded" position, but it seems only the Anti-Gravity Chain is capable of maintaining it perfectly. In this context, we are referring not only to sagittal plane load but

35

also to bilateral load in all three planes. In other words, we seek to promote bilateral, static postural stability before that of more dynamic, unilateral activities such as walking and running.

- Neutralize joint biomechanics. Lingering joint mechanic disparities should be the focus once load has been established. In much the same way that joint mechanics can resolve themselves during the process of selecting a therapeutic exercise which was based first on load, establishing the ability to maintain load in standing posture may correct faulty joint mechanics automatically. Should faulty joint mechanics persist, this is the appropriate phase in which to address them.

- Posturally Challenge and Reinforce function. In this final phase of postural therapy, the Anti-Gravity Chain is strengthened through even higher levels of demand. This is the phase in which heavy-demand strength training and athletics can be incorporated as a method of presenting postural challenges as well as for the sake of pursuing one's desired activity in a functional way.

The timeframe for progression through these phases varies considerably from person to person. Age, training status, pain, injury history, AGKC metabolic and neurologic status, superficial muscle/compensatory strength status, degree of postural deviation, and other factors will all affect the speed with which one can move from one phase to the next.

Function and Evaluation of the Kinetic Chain

We have discussed the concept of strain distribution and how the Antigravity Kinetic Chain can promote efficient division of labor in load bearing. In static standing posture the Anti-Gravity muscles promote body positioning that minimizes required resistance to mechanical strain. Joint position equilibrium exists when each joint accepts an appropriate fraction of systemic torque, strain is minimized, and all body segments work within their limitations. When one voluntarily changes their position, the center of gravity moves and the moments about each joint are changed. The body must find a new strain-minimizing joint position equilibrium, which is optimal for that position. The AGKC is also the mechanism by which joints collectively adapt to new body positions to redistribute strain throughout the body. To be sure, skeletal mechanisms are intimately involved here; however, it is the muscles that ultimately determine the position of the bony levers.

A healthy kinetic chain allows for human posture to accomplish its goal in different positions. Strengthening or reestablishing this mechanism is critical in optimizing function and reducing the pain that arises when a particular body segment attempts to accommodate inordinate amounts of strain. This is one of the most fundamental objectives of postural therapy. Efficiently distributing strain is dependent upon primary stabilizer health and requires a pathway clear of fascial or articular restriction from head to toe. Just as postural deviations can be classified as dysfunctions or compensations, a broken kinetic chain can be classified as broken either by dysfunction or by compensation.

How can we assess whether the kinetic chain is operational? If it is not, what tells us whether dysfunction or compensation is to blame? As we mentioned, changing the position of a joint requires that other joints change position in kind if strain is to be minimized. We are interested in the body's ability to make these changes from head to toe, and from toe to head. Specifically, we want to observe a cascade of strain-minimizing events that occur throughout the body when one segment changes position. Moreover, we want to observe that these events occur from the top down, from the bottom up, and from both ends simultaneously. The BuserGreus Kinetic Chain Tests were developed to evaluate the phenomenon of strain minimizing events in standing posture in order to guide therapy.

The Tests: "Hands-on-Head," "Pigeon-Toed," and "Both."

When assessing the kinetic chain, the initial concern should be whether or not an intact chain is present. Once it is established that a chain reaction can be observed throughout the body, the direction of greatest strength should be determined. Other factors such as length, tension, excitability, and both metabolic and neural endurance are also noteworthy.

We begin with a top-down test, "Hands on Head," in which the subject interlaces her fingers behind her head. From here, she alternates pulling her elbows back and then bringing them together in front of her head. We are most interested in the transition from the elbows touching in front of her face to the fully flared-open position. The back and forth motion resets the joints so we can observe the chain reaction repeatedly in this opening phase of the test. As the elbows are pulled back as far as possible, the healthy kinetic chain will exhibit: scapular retraction; thoracic, lumbar, and pelvic extension; hip flexion as the ilia extend relative to the femoral head; mild internal femoral rotation; mild hyperextension and abduction at the knee; internal rotation of the tibia with a tendency for the feet to follow although, being grounded they will not. Keep in mind, when performing these tests you are looking for a functional shift in the correct direction. The end result may not be a perfectly statically positioned joint. These tests evaluate dynamic movement of the kinetic chain at each joint towards the correct direction, in the correct order, and bilaterally at the same time.

We can reverse the test and observe the same mechanics from the bottom-up, "Pigeon-Toed," by having the subject pigeon-toe her feet (with the toes touching and heels out, feet angled at approximately 45 degrees) and alternately bending and straightening her knees such that they touch and then separate into hyperextension. Here we are interested in what takes place as the knees transition from a bent/touching position into a position of full extension. Again, if the chain is intact we should observe the aforementioned joint mechanics all the way up to scapular retraction with the addition of cervical spine and head extension, only this time in reverse. If both the top-down and the bottom-up test results are strong—meaning the expected joint mechanics are observed—compare the tests to each other to identify which direction exhibits the strongest kinetic connection. That is, the direction in which the expected joint mechanics were the most pronounced.

Finally, both tests can be performed at once to observe how the kinetic chain reacts to simultaneous stimulus from both directions. For this "Both" test, the fingers are interlaced behind the head and the feet are pigeon-toed at the same time. The subject bends her knees and brings the elbows together as described, opening the arms and extending the knees at the same time. Assuming that the chain is again healthy, the same cascade of joint events should begin from both ends travelling toward each other to meet in the middle. Should a positive finding occur in this third test, it should again be compared to the other two with ranks assigned to determine the direction of greatest kinetic chain strength.

The findings of these directional tests have important implications for postural therapy. Should we observe the chain to be broken, the priority is to reconnect it (Priorities-of-Work, Step 2). In the case of a broken chain, strain cannot be distributed. This constitutes a breakdown in the function of Anti-Gravity equilibrium mechanisms, and therefore in dynamic posture, which can cause a downward spiral of pain and compensatory offsets. Additionally, traditional exercise or other therapies cannot be counted on to effect change throughout the body "holistically" as the mechanism by which this would normally occur is nonoperational. Before more in depth corrective work can be done, the break in the kinetic chain must be addressed. Locating the break is as simple as watching to see where the chain reaction stops in a given test. Once the location is identified, load, joint mechanics, and muscle facilitation/inhibition can be used to restore functional distribution of strain through the segments that failed the directional tests. The results of the Kinetic Chain Tests can also be useful for practitioners of other modalities by allowing them to make use of directionality. For example, a chiropractor may elect to adjust the sacroiliac joint before the atlanto-occipital joint, or vice versa, based on the direction of greatest kinetic chain strength.

As we mentioned, a break in the kinetic chain can occur as a result of postural muscle dysfunction, superficial muscle compensation, or both, as is often the case. The clue as to which is the case lies in static posture. If a client or patient exhibits the gravity-induced "collapsing tendency", you can be reasonably sure that postural muscle dysfunction or weakness is primarily at play. Alternatively, if you observe deviations from normal postural alignment in any plane that disagrees with the "collapsing tendency" of the skeleton, at least some compensation must be involved. In either case, the therapeutic intervention should still be guided by optimizing load, joint mechanics, and muscle

40

facilitation/inhibition to reestablish the connection. Additionally, in the case of a compensatory break in the kinetic chain, the actual superficial muscles involved can often be visually observed as contracting or fasciculating against the proper action of the chain of events. This makes the course of action quite clear to both the practitioner and the patient. Add arrows showing the postural deficiency

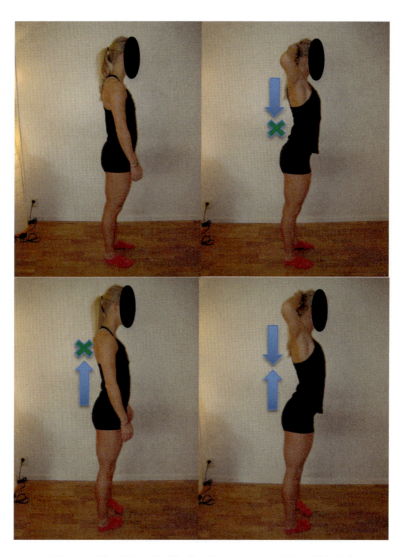

Figure 13: (Top Left) Static posture; (Top Right) "Hands-on-Head" Test: Notice the blue arrow indicating an intact kinetic chain until the level of the green "X"; (Bottom Left) "Pigeon-Toed" Test: Notice the blue arrow indicating an intact kinetic chain until the level of the green "X"; (Bottom Right) "Both" Test: Notice the blue arrows indicating the kinetic chain is reacting in the most normal or expected fashion during this test.

Chapter References

1.   Hodges P, Moseley GL, Gabrielsson A, Gandevia SC. Experimental muscle pain changes feedforward postural responses of the trunk muscles. Experimental brain research. Experimentelle Hirnforschung. Expérimentation cérébrale. 2003;151(2):262-271.

2.   Hodges P, Moseley GL. Pain and motor control of the lumbopelvic region: effect and possible mechanisms. Journal of electromyography and kinesiology : official journal of the International Society of Electrophysiological Kinesiology. 2003;13(4):361-370.

3.   Ervilha U, Farina D, Arendt-Nielsen L, Graven-Nielsen T. Experimental muscle pain changes motor control strategies in dynamic contractions. Experimental brain research. Experimentelle Hirnforschung. Expérimentation cérébrale. 2005;164(2):215-224.

How is this Therapeutic Model Different? Questions & Answers

In many respects, this model may be difficult to distinguish from similar models of exercise therapy. Like similar models, we emphasize the concepts of postural alignment, stabilization, kinetic chains, and the "core." And, we outline a method of applying these concepts through therapeutic exercise. Where our model differs, is in the understanding of 1) the collapsing tendency of the skeleton, and 2) the primary mechanism for resisting this collapsing tendency— the Anti-Gravity Kinetic Chain (AGKC). Some will see this distinction as subtle, but its implications for theory and practice are considerable. Most importantly, it allows us to differentiate between dysfunction and compensation. The ability to promote lasting, normal/optimal function rests upon this distinction.

What about the fact that research seems to support recruitment of mover-muscles such as the abdominals and erector spinae for mitigating pain and maintaining posture?

This kind of information is of great interest to our theoretical models and to our therapy. Many researchers have demonstrated the role of mover-muscles in various postural conditions and pain/injury/stability models.[1,2] We certainly don't discount these observations. The question is why do these observations arise? A cause-effect relationship between pain and muscle activity has been elusive,[3] but some relationship certainly exists.[4-7] Pain also interferes with postural stability.[8] Muscular inhibition may occur as an adaptive response to pain,[9] as a CNS measure to protect the body from further harm that may be caused by activity in painful muscles. Even if no apparent pain exists, weakness in mover-muscles could result from dysfunction of the muscles that stabilize the mover-muscles, the AGKC. Whatever the case may be, correlation alone does not indicate that these muscles account for mechanisms of pain/injury/instability, or that making them a therapeutic target will produce results.

Given our understanding of why these observations and results occur, our clinical impression is that the abdominals do not qualify for "postural-muscle" status. They fail the most important test of a primary stabilizing muscle—that is, they do not resist the effect of gravity. In fact, they exacerbate the effects of gravity, producing pelvic and trunk flexion, increased compressive forces throughout the spine and hips, and increased intradural pressure (as in a Valsalva maneuver). The abdominals also antagonize the diaphragm, our primary respiratory muscle, and a vital part of the fascial Anti-Gravity Chain. Notice how difficult breathing becomes when you perform the "drawing in" or "bracing" maneuvers with the abdominal muscles. Using the abdominals to "stabilize" the lumbar spine in static standing would require co-activation of the erectors, and would result in a great deal of unnecessary compression, regardless of whether co-activation is useful for stability during other movement tasks. The lumbar multifidi may be a better candidate for postural-muscle status, but do not feature quite as prominently, according to our theories, as the iliopsoas and quadratus lumborum. Compare the abdominals requirement for co-activation, to the psoas, which sits directly on the spine, maintaining lumbo-pelvic position, not only in static standing but also relative to the Line of Gravity and supporting a functional arch in the lower back without the need of co-activation. Remember, the curvature of the spine, maintained by the psoas, makes it far stronger than it would be as a straight rod.

Interestingly, variations on the abdominal "crunch" are a tool used frequently in our therapy. In certain cases they are an extremely appropriate exercise, which may explain some of the success reported by those who practice abdominal strength as a method of postural stabilization. The difference is the purpose for which abdominal exercises are applied. For us, the crunch has many uses, but strengthening the abdominals is the most seldom. Often, we use crunches to elicit reciprocal inhibition in the lumbar and lower thoracic erectors, muscles which are a frequent source of pain. We also use crunches with mildly kyphotic or thoracically "tight" clients to challenge the upper spine to maintain a functionally extended position. As a partial antagonist to the primary stabilizer chain, abdominal crunches are also effective in recruiting the stabilizing capacity of the AGKC. In all cases, an appropriate level of demand, proper positioning, and an understanding of the effects of any exercise is critical when applying crunches as part of any postural exercise regimen.

How can you say that the abdominals are not stabilizers? Any athlete will tell you that one cannot reach elite levels of competition without traditional core training programs.

To be clear, the abdominals can function as stabilizers. They do not appear adapted, however, to be primary stabilizers. The more traditional type of core strength (e.g. abdominal/erector strength), is likely relevant in athletic contexts. In any case, chronic pain and the functional limitations seen on a daily basis seem more likely to result from deficits in a deeper kind of strength. One that we suggest supports a more fundamental level of function. Of interest to the elite athlete, the basic functional strength we seek to develop can greatly enhance athletic performance.

Successful competition-level athletes do not necessarily exhibit greater integrity of the Anti-Gravity Kinetic Chain.

Variations in superficial muscle mass (i.e. any muscles other than those of the antigravity chain) will reflect the demands of their individual sports, but a tendency toward optimal load and joint mechanics can be observed across the entire spectrum. This is true of the marathon runner, the offensive lineman, and everything between. Returning to the question of the abdominals, think of it this way: the abdominals might assist with stabilization during sport-specific movement, but the primary stabilizer chain stabilizes the work of the abdominals. If you've experienced success training the "core" for stability, consider the exponential, catapulting affect one would find if they trained to stabilize the stabilizer-muscles.

As an example, consider the work involved in doing a push-up. The movement of the exercise involves the pectoralis major, deltoid, and triceps, among others. The abdominals, one could say, are engaged in a stability role, preventing lumbar hyperextension and anterior pelvic deviation, which would otherwise occur during the push-up position. The Anti-Gravity Kinetic Chain, however, stabilizes the work of the abdominals. Without involvement of the AGKC, abdominal engagement would result in posterior pelvic tilt and thoracic flexion, putting mover-muscles at a biomechanical disadvantage.

So if I activate the muscles of my anti-gravity chain I can improve posture and function while mitigating pain?

We would generally support that line of thought, but caution that effective postural therapy is not quite that simple. Targeting these muscles directly is a seldom approach, specific to our methodology. Moreover, the lack of direct internal antagonists to muscles of the AGKC makes volitional recruitment difficult at best. In any case, being stabilizers, the Anti-Gravity muscles must be recruited as such. Their role is not to move the bones to which they are attached, but to stabilize the bones against forces generated by other muscles, gravity, or elsewhere in the environment. Recruiting them in this capacity usually involves direct engagement of mover muscles so as to present the primary stabilizer chain with the challenge of maintaining a given bone position while work is being done. If our theories represent the science behind postural therapy, then eliciting appropriate stability challenges, through exercise, is the art of postural therapy. An effective exercise regimen will take into consideration what position(s) the subject must assume, which joint mechanics to promote, which muscle groups must be facilitated or inhibited, which contraindications are present, the intactness and preferred direction of the kinetic chain, and how to sequence exercises, while achieving the patient's predefined goal in the most efficient and effective manner.

So what kind of things should I be thinking about to improve posture?

The idea that thought plays a central role in postural alignment is somewhat misguided. While conscious thought may be able to override certain postural control mechanisms, maintenance of posture is primarily the duty of lower brain centers. Conscious processes, which allow for thought and volitional movement, are likely limited in their involvement. Postural alignment in all likelihood occurs automatically, leaving open the possibility of allocating attention to other, more specific tasks.[10] Conscious postural adjustments may be possible in the same way that one can choose to take a deep breath, but executive level brain functions need to be reserved for more complex matters. What's more, such conscious postural corrections will likely fail to recruit the proper muscles, those of the Anti-Gravity Chain, when making the desired adjustments.

These concepts are best understood through the works of Mabel Todd, an early student of somatic education. Her methods discussed body awareness but also respected the subconscious mechanisms that govern movement and stabilization.[11] Contemporary interpretations of the awareness concept, such as the idea that one's thoughts should be directed toward the intricacies of everyday movement, are probably not what the original teachers had in mind. The extent, to which we have our clients "think" through the process of correcting posture, is to think about relaxing compensatory, superficial, mover-muscles. Relaxation of this type may be a cortical brain phenomenon and can indirectly help shift the work of stabilization to the appropriate muscle groups.

There are therapies that attempt to correct pain or dysfunction through conscious movement re-education. Though this may work on a case-by-case basis, regardless of the mechanism by which it works, such an approach is not ideal. Reeducating movement without addressing static posture ignores the more pressing dysfunction. You might think of this as analogous to using a vehicle's steering column to compensate for a faulty vehicle alignment. In contrast, the therapy we practice aims to create an environment in which the optimal postural control strategy arises naturally. Movement is then corrected as a result, without the need for conscious movement re-education.

I have pain in my _____. Which exercises should I do?

This is a very common question for therapists of all kinds and unfortunately there is no universal answer. Many forms of therapy are based on protocols, which practitioners follow in the presence of given symptoms. In our experience, no two cases are alike regardless of how similar the presentations may be. Even if two clients complain of the exact same pain, it would be almost inconceivable for their postures, motor control strategies, stimulus profiles, and so on to be identical. Remember, the most important "symptom" in postural therapy is posture; pain tells us as much about what we cannot do than it does about what we can do. Musculoskeletal pain does not occur in a vacuum, it must be understood in the context of the postural or movement patterns that create it, as well as any traumatic sources that may be present. It is these postural or movement patterns which postural therapy seeks to address. A more prudent question would be "My posture and gait look like this, which exercises should I do?" Even then, however, the therapist would need to interview the client and consider all related factors, including pain, before an appropriate recommendation could be made.

Can you provide a detailed example of how you would apply load, joint mechanics, and muscle facilitation/inhibition to create an exercise that would pose a postural challenge to be met by the antigravity chain?

A very common recommendation in cases of low back pain involves lying on the ground with the lower legs placed on a chair or couch. The hips and knees are both bent to 90° with the lower legs (i.e. tibia/fibula) flush against the surface of the couch. The client relaxes and breathes from the diaphragm. This position has a reputation for being effective in relieving back pain and works the principles of load, joint mechanics, and muscle facilitation/inhibition.

The couch and ground assist the body in maintaining appropriate joint position. With this assistance, and the reduced anti-gravity demand found in the horizontal plane, the antigravity chain will assume the role of supporting joint position—even in many cases where severe postural deconditioning has occurred. Simply by using a position, we have created conditions in which the antigravity chain is more likely to arise as the most efficient stabilizer.

The joint mechanics of the position are fairly intricate. Hip and knee flexion facilitate the Anti-Gravity Chain by placing the hip and knee joints in a position where they are not made to resist gravity. Here, although hip flexion also couples with posterior pelvic tilt (i.e. pelvic flexion) and lumbar flexion, this challenges the Anti-Gravity Chain to engage and stabilize against lumbopelvic flexion. You might wonder, "Why not just make pelvic extension part of the position you select?" While this does work in certain scenarios, it has the potential to elicit compensation in the lumbar erectors, where strength is often deep-seeded and can be the source of pain in the lower back. In these cases, the subject would have to build up to more challenging positions of that type. At the same time, the posterior pelvic tilt and lumbar flexion cause a mechanical "whip" effect that travels superiorly along the spine and becomes thoracic extension, where antigravity facilitation is resumed. When dealing with posture and low back pain in particular, thoracic extension is very important, as the lumbar erectors will engage ever more forcefully to create this "whip" effect when thoracic extension is insufficient.

At the muscle level, several pathways are at work. First, the demand for compensatory muscular activity is reduced through assisted loading. This creates a loop wherein the Anti-Gravity Chain is further strengthened. This loop begins, when load facilitates the Anti-Gravity Chain and reduces the need for compensation. Next, the Anti-Gravity Chain is strengthened through positional stimulus. Then, the need for compensation is further reduced and the Anti-Gravity Chain gets more stimuli. In addition, the joint mechanics of hip and lumbar flexion inhibit the superficial back line, another of Myers' fascially continuous muscle chains. If we wanted to impose even more of a challenge on the Anti-Gravity Chain, we could simply introduce muscle actions that would aggravate the collapsing tendency of the skeleton, thereby causing the anti-collapsing muscles to engage in a stabilizing capacity. For instance, squeezing the gluteals would cause hip extension and/or squeezing the abdominals would cause a posterior pelvic tilt, requiring the iliopsoas and quadratus lumborum to engage for stability.

If you have used this position to achieve relief from lower back pain, you may have noticed the effects to be fleeting. If this was the case, it is likely that you were not placing enough demand on your postural system to force an adaptation that would transfer to meet the challenges of your lifestyle. For you, this position may only be part of a more comprehensive program to address your personal needs.

Chapter References

1.   Peate W, Bates G, Lunda K, Francis S, Bellamy K. Core strength: a new model for injury prediction and prevention. Journal of occupational medicine and toxicology (London, England). 2007;2.

2.   Willson JD, Dougherty CP, Ireland ML, Davis IM. Core stability and its relationship to lower extremity function and injury. Journal of the American Academy of Orthopaedic Surgeons. 2005;13(5):316-325.

3.   van Dieën JH, Selen LP, Cholewicki J. Trunk muscle activation in low-back pain patients, an analysis of the literature. Journal of Electromyography and Kinesiology Journal of Electromyography and Kinesiology. 2003;13(4):333-351.

4.   Ervilha U, Farina D, Arendt-Nielsen L, Graven-Nielsen T. Experimental muscle pain changes motor control strategies in dynamic contractions. Experimental brain research. Experimentelle Hirnforschung. Expérimentation cérébrale. 2005;164(2):215-224.

5.   Falla DL, Jull GA, Hodges PW. Patients with neck pain demonstrate reduced electromyographic activity of the deep cervical flexor muscles during performance of the craniocervical flexion test. Spine. 2004;29(19):2108-2114.

6.   Falla D, Jull G, Hodges P. Feedforward activity of the cervical flexor muscles during voluntary arm movements is delayed in chronic neck pain. Experimental brain research. 2004;157(1):43-48.

7.   Hodges P, Moseley GL, Gabrielsson A, Gandevia SC. Experimental muscle pain changes feedforward postural responses of the trunk muscles. Experimental brain research. Experimentelle Hirnforschung. Expérimentation cérébrale. 2003;151(2):262-271.

8.   Hirata RP, Ervilha UF, Arendt-Nielsen L, Graven-Nielsen T. Experimental muscle pain challenges the postural stability during quiet stance and unexpected

posture perturbation. The Journal of Pain. 2011;12(8):911-919.

9.   Lund JP, Donga R, Widmer CG, Stohler CS. The pain-adaptation model: a discussion of the relationship between chronic musculoskeletal pain and motor activity. Canadian journal of physiology and pharmacology. 1991;69(5):683-694.

10.   Schmidt RA, Lee T. Motor Control and Learning: A Behavioral Emphasis. 4th ed: Human kinetics; 1988.

11.   Todd ME. The thinking body. Dance horizons New York; 1975.

Made in the USA
San Bernardino, CA
13 August 2016